Breast cancer and prevention management

Table of contents

Introduction

Breast cancer is a disease that affects millions of people worldwide, and its impact can be devastating. Whether you have been diagnosed with breast cancer or are looking to take preventative measures, this book is here to guide you every step of the way. By providing you with the latest information on prevention and treatment options, "Breast Cancer Prevention and Management" offers a comprehensive approach to prevention and managing this disease. With expert advice from medical professionals, survivors, and caregivers, this book will inspire and empower you to take control of your health and make informed decisions about your care. Whether you are a patient, caregiver, or simply someone who wants to learn more about breast cancer, this book is a valuable resource for anyone looking to prevent and manage this disease. So let's begin this journey together and take the first step towards a healthier and happier future

Helpful Quotes on cancer prevention

"The best defense against cancer is to prevent it." - Dr. Harold Freeman

"Cancer prevention should be the cornerstone of any comprehensive cancer control plan." - Dr. Otis Brawley

"Prevention is better than cure." - Desiderius Erasmus

"Cancer can be prevented through healthy lifestyle choices and early detection." - Dr. David Agus

"The most important thing you can do to prevent cancer is to quit smoking." - Dr. Neal D. Barnard

"Cancer prevention is not just a slogan, it's a lifestyle." - Dr. David Servan-Schreiber

"The best way to prevent cancer is through a healthy diet and regular exercise." - Dr. David Katz

"Cancer prevention is everyone's responsibility." - Dr. David Satcher

"Cancer prevention requires a multi-faceted approach, including education, screening, and lifestyle changes." - Dr. Elizabeth Platz.

Breast cancer prevention advice

Breast cancer is a complex disease with many risk factors, some of which are beyond our control, such as genetics and age. However, there are some lifestyle changes you can make to reduce your risk of developing breast cancer. Here are some tips.

- Maintain a healthy weight: Being overweight or obese increases your risk of breast cancer, especially after menopause. So, maintaining a healthy weight through a balanced diet and regular exercise can help reduce your risk.

- Exercise regularly: Regular exercise, such as brisk walking or jogging, can help reduce your risk of breast cancer. Aim for at least 150 minutes of moderate-intensity exercise or 75 minutes of vigorous-intensity exercise per week.

- Limit alcohol intake: Drinking alcohol increases your risk of breast cancer. Limiting alcohol intake to no more than one drink per day can help reduce your risk.

- Quit smoking: Smoking has been linked to an increased risk of breast cancer. Quitting smoking can reduce your risk of not only breast cancer but other types of cancer and diseases.

- Breastfeed if possible: Breastfeeding can reduce your risk of breast cancer, especially if you breastfeed for at least one year.

- Get screened regularly: Early detection is key to treating breast cancer successfully. Women over 40 should have a mammogram every one to two years, or as recommended by their healthcare provider.

- Know your family history: If you have a family history of breast cancer, talk to your healthcare provider about your risk and whether additional screening or genetic testing is recommended.

Remember, these tips are not a guarantee against breast cancer, but they can help reduce your risk and improve your overall health.

Breast Cancer Prevention Through Diet and Food

Breast cancer is a serious health concern that affects many women around the world. While there are several factors that can increase your risk of developing breast cancer, such as genetics, family history, and age, there are also some dietary and lifestyle choices that can help reduce your risk. Below are some foods and diets that you can consider incorporating daily, into your regular routine to prevent breast cancer.

- Mediterranean diet: The Mediterranean diet is rich in fruits, vegetables, whole grains, and healthy fats such as olive oil, nuts, and fish. Studies have shown that following a Mediterranean-style diet may reduce the risk of breast cancer.

- Cruciferous vegetables: Vegetables like broccoli, cauliflower, kale, and Brussels sprouts contain compounds that can help reduce the risk of breast cancer.

- Fruits: Fruits such as berries, citrus fruits, and pomegranates are rich in antioxidants and other compounds that can help prevent breast cancer.

- Omega-3 fatty acids: Fish, nuts, and seeds are rich in omega-3 fatty acids, which have been shown to help prevent breast cancer.

- Green tea: Green tea is rich in antioxidants and has been shown to have anti-cancer properties, including the ability to help prevent breast cancer.

- Limit alcohol consumption: This comes as a caution. Women who drink alcohol regularly are at a higher risk of developing breast cancer. To reduce your risk, limit your alcohol consumption to no more than one drink per day, if you must drink.

- Maintain a healthy weight: Being overweight or obese can increase the risk of breast cancer, so maintaining a healthy weight through a balanced diet and regular exercise is important.

In a nutshell, a healthy diet and lifestyle that includes plenty of fruits, vegetables, whole grains, healthy fats, and lean protein, along with regular exercise, can help reduce your risk of breast cancer.

Breast Cancer Management Strategies

Breast cancer management requires a comprehensive approach that involves a combination of different treatment modalities, such as surgery, radiation therapy, chemotherapy, and targeted therapy. Some known tips to manage breast cancer are explained below.

- Seek expert medical advice: Breast cancer management requires the input of a team of medical professionals, including an oncologist, a surgeon, a radiation oncologist, and a pathologist. It is important to seek expert medical advice to ensure that you receive the best possible care.

- Learn about your breast cancer: Understanding the type, stage, and characteristics of your breast cancer is important in developing a personalized treatment plan. Talk to your medical team and research the latest information on breast cancer treatments and research.

- Consider all treatment options: There are many different treatment options available for breast cancer, including surgery, radiation therapy, chemotherapy, targeted therapy, and hormone therapy. Discuss all the available treatment options with your medical team to determine the best approach for you.

- Take care of your mental and emotional health: A breast cancer diagnosis can be overwhelming and stressful. It is important to prioritize your mental and emotional well-being. Consider seeing a therapist or joining a support group to help you cope with the emotional impact of breast cancer.

- Maintain a healthy lifestyle: A healthy lifestyle can help support your body through the breast cancer treatment process. Eat a balanced diet, exercise regularly, get enough sleep, and avoid smoking and excessive alcohol consumption.

- Communicate with your medical team: Effective communication with your medical team is crucial to ensure that you receive the best possible care. Make sure to ask questions, share concerns, and discuss any side effects or symptoms you may be experiencing.

- Stay informed about your follow-up care: Breast cancer treatment is often ongoing, and it is important to stay informed about your follow-up care. Attend all scheduled appointments, follow your medical team's recommendations for ongoing monitoring and testing, and report any new symptoms or concerns promptly.

A survivor's firsthand knowledge of cancer management.

It was learned that the cancer was at Stage 3, and that it was estrogen receptor (ER) positive, progesterone receptor (PR) positive and growth factor (HER2) negative. As a result, her treatment plan included chemotherapy, followed by surgery and radiation.

"I was so relieved once I knew what stage the cancer was and what my treatment would be," she said. "I was like, OK, let's do this."

When I went for chemo, there were three nurses there. They treated me like we were sisters. I love them a lot," she said.

Once she finished chemotherapy, she had a big decision to make. Surgical oncologist Jamie Rand, M.D., assistant professor in the Division of Breast Surgery at City of Hope in Duarte, explained in detail her choices — she could have a mastectomy to remove the entire breast or a lumpectomy to remove only the cancer.

She chose the lumpectomy, which was followed by adjuvant radiation.

Today, she has been in remission for more than a year — and to help keep it that way, she continues to take two estrogen-blocking drugs, tamoxifen and Zoladex.

The origin of her cancer wasn't genetic, she believes the cause might have been linked to her lifestyle. She was overweight, and her diet included too much sugar and foods with chemical additives.

"After my diagnosis, we changed our way of living," She said. "The whole family started eating organic food, a lot more veggies without preservatives, and no sugar."

I sincerely want to note here that your lifestyle and eating habits can influence your freedom from breast cancer. Avoiding much intake of sugar and sugary junks plus food with chemical additives, will go a long way to guide you against breast cancer.

Breast Cancer Prevention: Medicinal Herbs

There are several medicinal herbs that have been traditionally used to prevent breast cancer, and some of them have also been studied for their potential anti-cancer properties. However, it's important to note that, despite these herbs being medicinally useful against cancer, there is limited scientific evidence to support the use of herbs for cancer prevention, and it's always best to consult with a healthcare professional before using any herbal remedies.

Below are some herbs that have been traditionally used to prevent breast cancer.

- Turmeric: This herb is commonly used in Indian cuisine and is known for its anti-inflammatory properties. Some studies suggest that curcumin, the active compound in turmeric, may help prevent breast cancer.

- Green tea: Green tea contains a type of polyphenol called catechins, which have been shown to have anti-cancer properties. Some studies suggest that drinking green tea may help reduce the risk of breast cancer.

- Garlic: Garlic has been used for medicinal purposes for centuries and has been shown to have anti-cancer properties. Some studies suggest that consuming garlic may help prevent breast cancer.

- Ginger: Ginger is known for its anti-inflammatory and anti-cancer properties. Some studies suggest that ginger may help prevent breast cancer.

- Milk thistle: Milk thistle is a plant that has been traditionally used for liver problems, but it also has anti-cancer properties. Some studies suggest that milk thistle may help prevent breast cancer.

- Onion: Onion is also a known herb that is important to cancer prevention. It has anti-cancerous properties and l advice you should take it raw as frequently as possible.

It's crucial to remember that, while these herbs may have significant health advantages, including anti-cancer properties, they are not a replacement for medical therapy. It is always recommended to talk with a healthcare practitioner if you are concerned about your risk of breast cancer.

The herbs described above should be used and consumed on a daily basis. This will help maximize their effectiveness against malignant tumors and growth.